The Evaluator's Cookbook

The Evaluator's Cookbook

Exercises for participatory evaluation with children and young people

Angus McCabe and Katrice Horsley

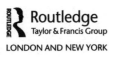

Routledge
Taylor & Francis Group

LONDON AND NEW YORK

First published 2008 by Routledge
2 Park Square, Milton Park, Abingdon, Oxon OX14 4RN

Simultaneously published in the USA and Canada
by Routledge
270 Madison Avenue, New York, NY 10016

Routledge is an imprint of the Taylor & Francis Group, an informa business

© 2008 Angus McCabe & Katrice Horsley

Typeset in Myriad and New Baskerville by the authors
Printed and bound in Great Britain by Bell & Bain Ltd, Glasgow

British Library Cataloguing in Publication Data
A catalogue record for this book is available from the British Library

Library of Congress Cataloging-in-Publication Data
McCabe, Angus.
   The evaluator's cookbook : exercises for partipatory evaluation with children and young people / Angus McCabe and Katrice Horsley.
      p.cm.
   ISBN 978–0–415–45341–7
   1. Social work education. 2. Social workers—In-service training. 3. Social work with children—Study and teaching. 4. Family social work—Study and teaching. 5. Social work with youth—Study and teaching. 6. Social service—Study and teaching. I. Horsley, Katrice. II. Title.
   HV11.5.M39 2008
   362.7—dc22   2007048547

ISBN 10: 0-415-45341-0 (pbk)
ISBN 10: 0-203-92687-0 (ebk)
ISBN 13: 978-0-415-45341-7 (pbk)
ISBN 13: 978-0-203-92687-1 (ebk)

Contents

Foreword

With this Cookbook in hand, it will be difficult for anyone to argue that children cannot be engaged creatively with services. There are lots of ideas, and the 'ingredients' at the end and the associated website make it easy to get started. Some of the recipes could easily be adapted for adults too.

Professor Marilyn Taylor, University of the West of England

Introduction

Why an Evaluator's Cookbook?

The Evaluator's Cookbook was developed through the National Evaluation of the Children's Fund (NECF) at the University of Birmingham. Funded by the Department for Education and Skills, NECF undertook an evaluation of the Children's Fund (England) between 2003 and 2006 which explored the impact of the programme's preventative services on the lives of children and young people (aged 5–13).

Early in the evaluation, one common theme emerged. Practitioners, participation workers, evaluators and academics all commented on the difficulties of undertaking evaluation with younger children and the lack of resources for doing so.

As a result, much of the evaluation activity around the Children's Fund, preventative services for children and families more generally, has focused on seeking the views of older children (aged 9 plus), parents, carers or professionals involved in delivering services.

The methods used to gather children's views, feelings and thoughts about their communities and the services they receive have often tended to be very traditional: questionnaires, surveys, structured interviews, focus groups and so forth. However, such techniques often assume that participants in research and evaluation have well developed literacy or numeracy skills and do not fully acknowledge the fact that all of us, whether adults or children, express and like to convey information about ourselves and our world in different ways; through song, photographs, painting, story telling and other media.

The Cookbook therefore offers:

- a series of arts and activity based evaluation exercises

- suggestions on visual means of presenting findings

- interactive, information technology based, resources

Further, it acknowledges that accepted approaches to research and evaluation are not to 'everyone's taste.' Using different 'recipes' is essential to reach different groups – in different ways which appeal to their 'sense of taste'. Being formally questioned can be a frightening experience – particularly those who lack self confidence. Some may associate interviews and questionnaires with being tested or negative experiences of trying to access, or actually use, services for children and families. For others, some research methods can be seen as imposing adult views, interpretations and values on the experiences of children and young people.

Adopting more arts, crafts and multi-media research and evaluation methods may allow children and adults to express themselves both in more creative and, by using media that people feel comfortable or familiar with, in more expansive and honest ways.

Thus, research and evaluation may engage more effectively with those groups often referred to as 'hard to reach' – and, hopefully, become an experience which is enjoyed by all those participating in the process, rather than being something alien and imposed.

The aim of the Evaluator's Cookbook then is not to replace tried and tested research methods. It is there to add to the range of techniques available to academics, practitioners and others as well as introduce new ways of gathering information and help make evaluation a creative, as well as scientific, process.

Introduction

Who is the Cookbook for?

The Evaluator's Cookbook is intended primarily as a resource for those:
- researching the experiences of children, young people and their families
- evaluating education or other services for children and young people
- practitioners, teachers and trainers wishing to gather the views of young people on a particular event or intervention
- working to promote the participation of children and young people in decision making

However, the recipes in the Cookbook are designed to be flexible and have been used in a range of settings and for different purposes with adults as well as children and young people. For example, Heraldic Banners, page 26, can be adapted to help organisations create a visual picture of their vision and purpose. Pockets, page 51, has proved a useful tool in gathering people's ideas (either as drawings, photographs or text) for public consultations – 'how can we improve our neighbourhood?' The Tree, page 51, has been useful in helping agencies think about how they can improve their services for users, with giant ones being placed in foyers and users' responses being placed upon them.

The recipes in the Cookbook are designed to be inclusive and have been used with disabled children, adults and people with a learning disability. The Emotion Tree in the Virtual Cookbook, page 52, (www.nemisys.uk.com/cookbook) was specifically designed for children with Asperger's Syndrome – or those who may find it difficult to express ideas and feelings in a group setting. Stretching the Point has been used successfully in Special Needs settings, with elastics tied to wheelchairs as well as being held by others.

About the Cookbook

The Cookbook is divided into three main sections:

Starters
These are short 'warm-up' exercises which can be used to generate initial evaluation ideas and issues as well as setting a framework for actually evaluating individual sessions with participants.

Main Courses
These are more substantial exercises, aimed at providing children and young people with opportunities to creatively explore the issues in their lives and generate evaluation information.

Puddings
These are again shorter exercises to 'round off' and evaluate sessions with participants.

The final sections add:

- a series of exercises suggesting creative ways of presenting data – both immediately to participants in a particular event or to a wider audience interested in the findings of an evaluation or consultative exercise.
- interactive technology based approaches to gathering and presenting information. These resources are free and can be viewed and downloaded by visiting www.nemisys.uk.com/cookbook.
- templates for key exercises (for example Locks and Keys, page 9) which can be photocopied for use.

Using the recipes

Each page of the Cookbook contains a recipe which gives:

- The **name** of the exercise
- Suggestions on:

The **preparation time** required

The **time taken** to run the exercise

The **energy levels** involved
8 – highly physical;
3 – quieter/more reflective

The maximum **number of participants** (quantity)

- The **ingredients** (equipment/materials required)
- The **methods** (instructions for use)

Examples of how each recipe has been used are also included. However, the Cookbook is there to be adapted according to the needs of the groups being worked with and to stimulate other ideas for creative approaches to evaluation, research and consultation. They can be used on a one-to-one basis, with small groups, in a whole classroom setting or, indeed, in large public events. Enjoy, use or amend!

What will the Cookbook tell us?

Most of the exercises in the Cookbook are designed to be part of the process of qualitative research and evaluation. They can tell us what children, young people and their families think and feel about their community, the services they use or the issues they face.

Others may be helpful in yielding quantitative data. For example, the O-meters (Interactive Cookbook: www.nemisys.uk.com/cookbook) allow for an aggregate 'score' of the views of children about the services they receive generally or to gather their views on a one-off session. Stretching the Point, page 13, can equally be used to establish numerical patterns – x number of people thought this, y number felt that . . .

Arts based methods are powerful tools for seeking peoples ideas and views. They do not, necessarily, tell evaluators or others why people hold a particular view or why they believe something. Combining the recipes in the Cookbook with more traditional research techniques can therefore be useful – for example using each exercise as a starting point for discussions using semi-structured interview questions:

- 'That's an interesting drawing/picture . . . could you tell me more about that?'
- 'So what you have done is . . . why do you feel that way? Why do you think that . . . ?'

Again, a note of caution. As with any objective research, the interpretation of the professional should not get in the way of the message and meaning conveyed by the evaluation participant , whether they be an adult or, particularly, a child.

Thinking about the recipes

The Evaluator's Cookbook offers a menu of participatory research and evaluation exercises. Each can be 'mixed and matched' through using particular 'starters', 'main courses' and 'puddings'. But techniques are only as good as the overall process and contexts they are placed within. Before using the recipes, it is important to consider a range of issues. For example:

● who is the audience for the findings from our research and evaluation? Will they be receptive to arts-based presentations of information – or is what they require more statistical data?

● if we present findings as pictures, drawings or stories – will they be taken seriously by a wider/adult audience?

● are the techniques we are using appropriate for the groups we are working with – in terms of age, the level of literacy required, participants' comfort in using different media for expression?

● many of the Cookbook's exercises rely on using junk materials – old scraps of materials, discarded objects, etc. Using some materials in some cultural settings may be inappropriate (e.g. leather). Colours have different meanings in different cultures. Are we sufficiently aware of these issues before using a particular exercise?

● using drawings, stories and other arts-based approaches – although participatory and hopefully enjoyable – can raise some very personal and painful issues for children and adults. In testing the materials included in the Cookbook, these issues have included uncovering instances of bullying, abuse and dealing with bereavement. Are we prepared to acknowledge and address these issues in the evaluation/research process? How are we going to respond?

Participatory evaluation can be seen as an 'easy option' – one which lacks the rigour of more traditional academic methods. This is not the case. Just as much thought needs to be dedicated to planning and analysing participatory approaches and the information they generate as is required in designing questionnaires, interview schedules and survey samples. Their advantage may be, when used appropriately and as part of a wider process, that arts and multi media methods can be a powerful statement about our values as evaluators and re-balance the power relationship between the professional researcher/consultant and 'research subjects'.

Acknowledgements

The authors would like to thank:

● The Department for Education and Skills, England (now the Department for Children, Schools and Families) who encouraged and financially supported the development of an earlier version of The Evaluator's Cookbook as part of the National Evaluation of the Children's Fund.

● Coventry Children's Fund for allowing the use of 'Picture This'.

● Nemisys Enterprises Ltd for the design and layout of the Cookbook and for hosting the interactive 'Virtual Cookbook'.

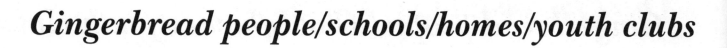

Gingerbread people/schools/homes/youth clubs

Ingredients

- Laminated line drawings of the subject you want to explore. One for each participant. (Remember, as they are laminated they can be used again)

- OHP pens

Method

- Ask participants to draw/write inside the image all the feelings they have about what it is really like, or should be like
- Ask them to draw outside the image how it appears to others – e.g. School – outside, a place where you learn, make friends, get supported. Inside, a noisy place, where you get jostled and you feel alone

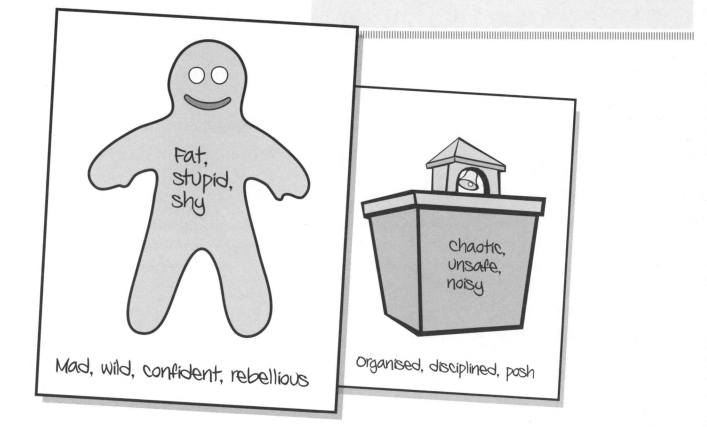

Fat, stupid, shy

Mad, wild, confident, rebellious

chaotic, unsafe, noisy

Organised, disciplined, posh

Preparation time
30 minutes

Cooking time
15–20 minutes

Energy level
6

Quantity
30

5

Gingerbread people/schools/homes/youth clubs

This exercise can be used and adapted for a range of ages and abilities and is especially suitable for younger children.

If participants are unable to write, images can be drawn or pictures from magazines can be cut out and placed on the laminates.

Try and keep the laminates large enough for participants to place images on, especially if you want a group response.

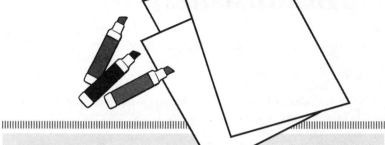

STARTER

Hands/scales

Ingredients

- OHP projectors
- Acetates
- OHP pens in different colours

Method

- Choose a subject you wish to explore, e.g. youth service, school environment
- Ask participants to draw a set of old fashioned scales or to draw around their hands
- On one side of the scales, or in one hand, draw images or write words depicting positive aspects of the subject
- On the other side of the scales or on the other hand draw images or write words that depict the negative aspects of the subject
- Project the images onto a wall or onto each other (see the presentation section at the end of this book)
- Discuss

NB Katrice Horsley would like to acknowledge Jim Morris for the hands idea in this exercise

Preparation time
Collection of equipment

Cooking time
30 minutes

Energy level
7

Quantity
10

Hands/scales

This has been successful with young people (12–16 years) and adults. Voice work can be used to supplement it by inviting individuals to name a positive aspect and asking the rest of the group to repeat this.

Other images can be used such as shut doors and open doors.

Locks and keys

Ingredients

- Large white images of padlocks that are laminated
- Large white images of keys that are laminated
- Big white clouds that are laminated
- OHP pens

Method

- Split into groups of about 4–6, each participant to have one key, cloud and lock each
- Ask participants to think of an objective they wish to achieve, e.g. attend school more regularly and write/draw it on a cloud
- Ask participants in the groups to ask them what stops them achieving this and draw/write it on the padlocks
- Next ask them to identify a way of overcoming this and draw/write it on the key
- The padlock, key and cloud should form a path/line
- Ask participants to discuss their findings in small groups. You may want to photograph the findings as a record
- Templates for this exercise are available in the 'Ingredients' section of the Cookbook

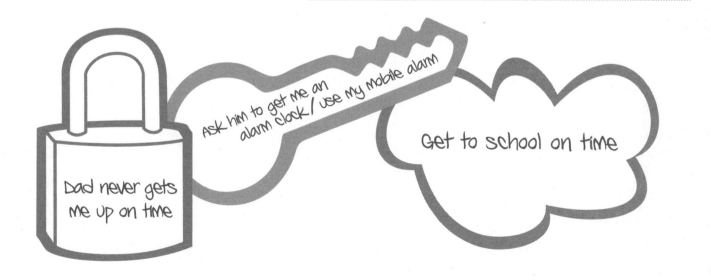

Dad never gets me up on time

Ask him to get me an alarm clock / use my mobile alarm

Get to school on time

Preparation time
30 minutes

Cooking time
30 minutes

Energy level
7

Quantity
30, to be used in groups

Locks and keys

This exercise has been used in a range of ways with most age groups, especially to look at the issue of accessing a service.

As an adaptation an image of the service can be provided, e.g. photograph of a school, instead of the cloud. Participants can then be invited to draw images of what prevents them from attending on the locks, and possible solutions on the keys.

Machines

Method

Ingredients

None needed

- Identify the subject you wish to explore – e.g. school, home, hospital
- Ask participants to each think of a phrase that reflects this subject for them – e.g. Hospital – 'scary and big'. They could also choose a phrase they hear a lot in this environment – e.g. Hospital – 'take a seat please'
- Ask them to each think of this phrase and make it more rhythmic
- In a circle ask them all to repeat their own phrase. This should last for about 30 cacophonous seconds!
- Ask them each to then add a movement to their phrase – perhaps just bending up and down, or moving their head or something more adventurous
- In a circle get them to repeat their phrases and make their movements, again all of them doing this at the same time. This will ensure that no one feels particularly exposed

- Now allocate them numbers and ask them to make their movement and sound in sequence around the circle, each taking turns
- Invite them to become attached to each other by holding hands, touching elbows, etc and form a 'machine'
- Ask them to repeat their movements and phrases in sequence again, remembering their numbers to get the sequence right. Let this process happen for a minute or so to enable all of the phrases to be heard
- You can record the results onto video or audio tape and it will provide a baseline assessment of their reactions/experiences towards the chosen subject. The exercise can be repeated later on to see if participants have experienced any changes in the subject area

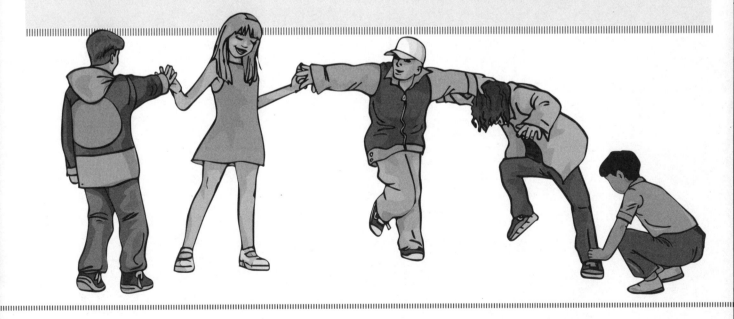

Preparation time
Nil

Cooking time
15 minutes

Energy level
8

Quantity
15–20 for one big batch, more if you break it into smaller ones

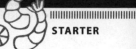

Machines

This exercise tends to work better with children between 8–12 years. Some older children can find it a little 'exposing' unless it is introduced in the right way.

If physical contact is an issue participants can be joined by string or sticks and for those with limited mobility it can also be done whilst sitting down.

STARTER

Stretching the point

Ingredients

- 1½ metre sections of sewing elastic, about three pieces for each participant
- Card (A4)
- Felt tip pens

Method

- Identify the subject you want to explore and then ask participants to identify what they like/dislike about it or would wish to change
- Ask participants to draw/write a selection of these (about 4–5 at a time) on pieces of card
- Choose people to hold the cards
- The other participants must hold on to the ends of their pieces of elastic. A command must be called out, e.g. 'What do you like most about school?'. Participants must then give the free ends of their elastics to card holders in order to cast a vote for their top three preferences. In this way a giant human and elastic web will be made as well as preferences identified
- Ask card holders to tally up how many elastics they are holding at the end of each command and note these down for later discussion
- Be careful when letting go of the elastics – always ask card holders to keep them down below waist level before letting go!

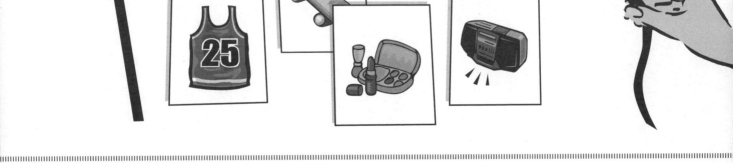

Preparation time
Purchasing lots of elastic!

Cooking time
15 minutes to ½ hour

Energy level
10

Quantity
15–25

Stretching the point

This has proved to be one of the most enjoyable evaluation techniques! It can be used very successfully with all age ranges. If the elastic proves to be a risk, ribbon or string can also be used.

STARTER

Stretching the point boards *(part 1)*

Ingredients

- ½ inch plyboard about 80 cm x 60 cm
- Drill
- Pieces of elastic (2–3 for each member of the group) long enough to reach from the centre of the board to the edges. Better if it is tubular elastic
- Sticky Velcro, both 'male' and 'female', enough to go around the circumference of the board
- Paint
- Images of indicators
- Images of the subjects you wish to explore
- Post-its

Method

- Make a series of holes in the centre of the board – 2–3 for each participant. They should be small enough to just thread the elastic through
- Paint the board and leave it to dry
- Attach the one strip of Velcro (either the male or the female) around the edge of the board to make a frame – about 5 cm deep
- Thread sections of elastic through the holes so that the ends are at the front of the board and they are long enough to reach the edges. (You can either have one piece of elastic per hole and knot it at the back or one piece of elastic through two holes and knot it at the front)
- On the edge of each piece of elastic, fold small squares of Velcro (the opposite type to the border so it will stick!)
- Place images of the subjects you wish to investigate at the edges of the board (usually a maximum of 4, one for each side). These can be temporarily secured with Blue Tac/Sellotape
- Give out a command – e.g. What activity do you most like doing at your playcentre? And ask participants to stick two–three pieces of elastic onto the areas of the frame that contains the images of their 'votes'
- Ask them to write on Post-its why they made this choice and attach them to their elastic pieces
- Photographs can be taken and the results discussed. The boards can be re-used with other images to cover different subjects

Preparation time
2 hours

Cooking time
15 minutes

Energy level
5

Quantity
6 people per board,
depending on its size

Stretching the point boards *(part 2)*

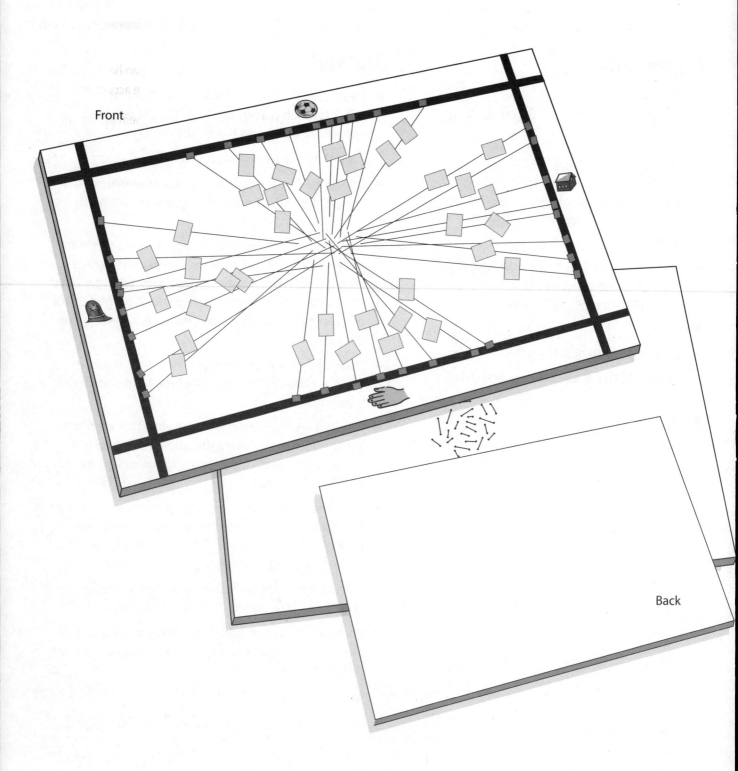

Front

Back

Preparation time
2 hours

Cooking time
15 minutes

Energy level
5

Quantity
6 people per board,
depending on its size

Stretching the point boards

Individual boards can be made from stiff card so that an ongoing evaluation can take place. Individuals can have images of what they need to achieve around the edges and then place their string upon it when they feel they have accomplished it.

Extra large ones can also be made for foyer areas and users of the organisation can be invited to utilise them as they leave the building.

Targets

Ingredients

- A1 mounting board – white
- Piece of string
- Drawing pin
- Pens
- Paints
- Post-its
- Images of indicators
- Digital camera

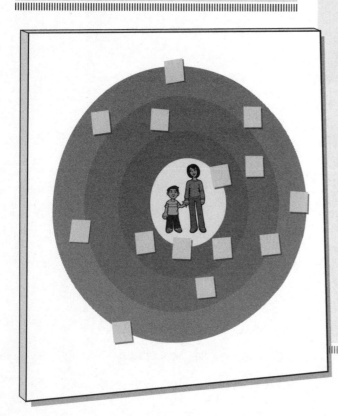

Method

- Identify the subject you want to explore

- Onto the board draw a series of about 4–5 concentric circles, about 5 cm wide

- Paint the circles in different colours to produce a 'target'

- Choose the subject area or issue that you wish the board to represent. e.g. Where do you feel most valued/most listened to/most safe?

- Ask participants to place Post-its on the board in response to these. The responses nearest the centre of the board represent the most, those further away, the least. They can draw images or if you wish you could have a selection to hand that they can use

- The targets can be used to elicit a variety of other information too, such as what is most or least liked about a subject, what equipment they would like to see in a certain environment, etc. The possibilities are endless!

- Discuss findings and take photos for reference

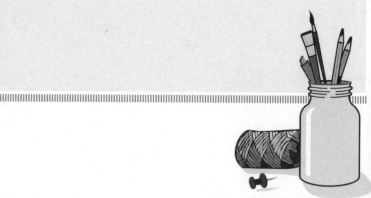

Preparation time
About 1½ hours

Cooking time
15 minutes

Energy level
5

Quantity
About 5 people per target

Targets

This has been used as a great alternative to the standard 1–5 questionnaire. (1 being strongly disagree, 5 strongly agree.) That usually requires a reading level of 12 to understand! If you ensure there are five rings in the target, the same information can be gathered from children and people who may not have sufficient literacy skills or not have enough English to fully understand a written questionnaire.

A space of our own

Ingredients

- Shoe boxes (one for each participant or for a group of about 4)
- Pipe cleaners
- Plasticine
- Bits of card and coloured paper
- Scissors
- Glue
- Colouring crayons/felt tips

Method

- Identify the subject you wish to explore, e.g. school, hospital, their home
- Ask children to use the materials to build a 3-dimensional model of how they would like the subject area to be
- Ask them to label their models, provide clocks to show the amount of time they like to spend there, menus to show what food they would like to eat (if applicable), mini music CDs to show what music they may want to listen to, etc
- Ask them to share their spaces with the rest of the group and explain their reasons for designing them this way
- Discuss the findings

Preparation time
30 minutes

Cooking time
30–45 minutes

Energy level
5

Quantity
Up to 20

A space of our own

Whilst this was primarily designed for children it has also been used very successfully with adults to explore their responses to a service. It is important to ensure that materials used are attractive to both genders; these can include clay, wood, wire, boxes, as well as fabrics and stickers, etc.

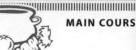

CD covers

Ingredients

- Blank CD covers
- Glue
- Pens
- Scissors
- Range of magazines/images that appeal to the group
- Card cut to fit into the CD covers – two pieces per participant

Method

- Ask participants to think of a subject they would like to explore – perhaps themselves, their education?
- Ask them to make a collage image of how the subject appears to others on a piece of card (Image 1)
- Ask them to create a collage image of their personal experience of the subject (Image 2)
- Ask them to think of acknowledgements – such as you find in CD covers – do they have any they would like to write? If so ask them to write them on the back of Image 2
- Do they have any lyrics/words that link into the subject? Can they make any up? They should place these on the back of Image 1
- They should place Image 1 in a CD case to make the front cover. Image 2 should be placed so that the acknowledgements are placed outward to make the back cover – the image being on the inside
- Invite the participants to share their personal CDs with the rest of the group

Preparation time
Collection of inclusive collage materials

Cooking time
30 minutes

Energy level
5

Quantity
Works better with smaller groups of older children

CD covers

This exercise was found to be particularly successful with teenagers. It is really a variant of 'Gingerbread People.'

It can be adapted so that 'collections' are made that cover different areas of a service, such as access, range of activities, etc.

Collages

Ingredients

- A selection of magazines, images and catalogues that cover the area you wish to explore. Remember to be as inclusive as possible when choosing these images

- Glue

- Scissors

Method

- Ask participants to fold their paper in half

- Identify the area you wish to explore, e.g. health, school, particular services, etc

- Ask participants to cut out images of the subject as they experience it. They should stick these on one side of the card in any shape they wish

- Ask participants to imagine how they would like the area under discussion to be and stick images on the other half of the card

- This can be done in small groups or as an individual exercise

- Discuss findings

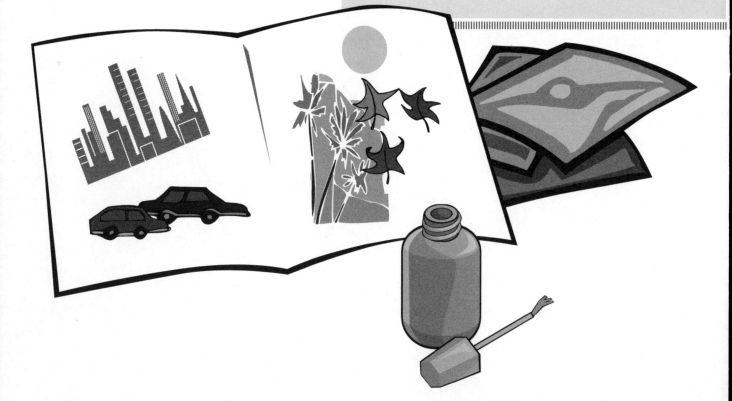

Preparation time
1–15 minutes

Cooking time
30 minutes

Energy level
4

Quantity
Up to 30

Collages

This again is an adaptation of 'Gingerbread People' but is a little more accessible to those who may have more limited fine motor skills and would experience problems with finely placing images within an outline.

Preprinted icons or images can be used if a more focused response is needed.

Heraldic banners

Ingredients

- Large pieces of canvas (if working in groups). Small pieces of canvas if working individually

- A range of fabrics, felt, cotton, etc

- Ribbon of varying thicknesses and colours

- Glue guns or Copydex

- Scissors

- Gaffer tape

- Pieces of dowling

- Images of heraldic design/banners to share

Method

- Cut the fabric into large/small banner shapes

- Identify the area you want to explore, e.g. school, health, access to services

- Ask participants to divide up their banner into sections and think about the area to be discussed. They should sketch some images from their ideas onto paper first

- Ask participants to design the banner based on their experience of the area in question. They may want to divide it into positives and negatives again

- They should use the fabrics and ribbons to make the design

- Ask participants to share their banners and what they symbolise with the rest of the group. Discuss

Preparation time
Material collection and cutting out of banners if desired

Cooking time
30 minutes for making banners, 30 minutes for discussion

Energy level
6

Quantity
Groups of 4 or individually – about 30

Heraldic banners

This has been a highly successful exercise for adults and children alike. It has been used to design Mission Statements, evaluate most enjoyed activities and explore personal responses to a service.

If time is limited, paper can be used and if time is not an issue Velcro could be used so that the finished result can be changed if so desired.

Masks

Ingredients

- Large A1 pieces of thin card, one for each participant
- Scraps of card
- Scissors
- Glue
- Tape
- Laminated speech bubbles if desired

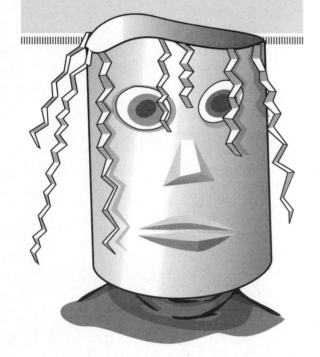

Method

- Ask participants to choose a shape for their head mask. Perhaps a curved top/straight top/asymmetric, etc

- Ask them to cut the top of the card (widthways)to the required shape

- They should then make the card into a giant cylinder that will fit over their heads and rest on their shoulders. This is the basis for the mask

- Ask participants to decorate the masks using pieces of card to create ears, eyes, eyebrows, noses, etc. It is very effective if you can score the card pieces to create a 3-dimensional effect

- Participants should identify a character for the mask, such as a health visitor, social worker, doctor, parent, etc

- Ask participants to think of a phrase that the character might be heard to say. They can put on the mask and say this to the rest of the group. Have the group repeat the phrase back

- Ask participants to think of a phrase that the character might really want to say. Repeat the above

- If participants do not wish to talk they can use the speech bubbles and have the group read them back

- Discuss findings

Preparation time
Just material collection

Cooking time
30 minutes to make masks,
30/45 minutes for use

Energy level
5

Quantity
Enough for about 20

Masks

This is suitable for children 6 years upwards. The masks can also be used to reflect how participants want a service to be or how a service makes them feel.

Mirrors to the future

Ingredients

- A selection of mirror tiles – one for each participant
- Thick corrugated card large enough to 'frame' the tiles and provide a back to the mirror. (About A4 size)
- A selection of images from magazines
- Spray paints or acrylics
- A selection of art materials, thick string, shells, card, sticks, etc
- Scissors
- PVA glue
- Masking tape and gaffer tape
- Small card/paper shapes (stars, squares, etc)
- Laminator (optional)

Method

- Ask participants to stick the mirror onto the backing card. They can tape around the edges if they wish as they will not be seen
- Ask them to cut out a wide frame to fit around the mirror and onto the backing board. If they are going to spray paint or paint the frame they should do that now, otherwise they may get the paint on the mirror
- Attach the frame and backing board together, with the mirror in the centre so that it is sandwiched between the two. Paint around the edges if needed using a brush or decorative tape
- Ask participants to think of where they would like to be in the future. Decorate around the frame with images that represent their desires
- Invite participants to share their mirror with the rest of the group
- Ask them to identify any obstacles that may prevent them realising their ambition and draw images of them onto one side of the small card shapes. Let them share these with the group if they wish
- Ask them to think of strategies for overcoming these obstacles and draw them on the reverse side of the card shapes, the group may want to offer suggestions too
- Hang the card pieces off the bottom of the mirrors

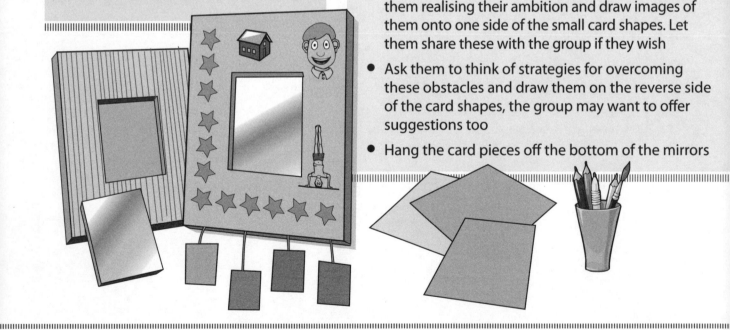

Preparation time	Cooking time	Energy level	Quantity
Collection of materials	1 hour–1 hour 30 minutes	3	Small groups of older children (10 upwards)

Mirrors to the future

The end result of this exercise is certainly worth the effort. The activity is suitable for 9 years upwards because of the health and safety element.

The mirrors can be re-used if desired with participants removing objectives when they have been met and hanging others that have been identified.

Puppets

Ingredients

- Thin coloured card, 2 pieces for each participant
- Bits of coloured paper
- Sticky tape
- Scissors

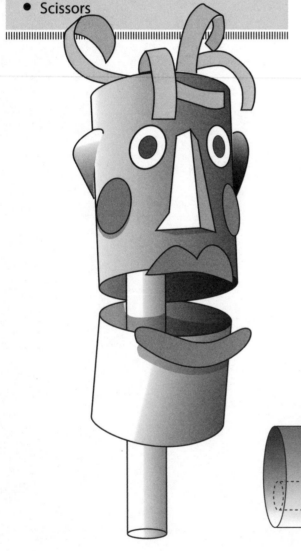

Method

- Ask participants to take one piece of card and form a wide tube, using the paper sideways. Tape the edges together. This is the head

- Cut off the lower third of this tube, this is the lower jaw

- Take the remaining piece of card and roll it into a narrow tube, longways – this will form the 'handle' of the puppet

- Place the handle into the head and jaw, make sure the taped join of the head is at the back. Attach the head to the handle with tape. Take the lower jaw and attach it back onto the head with a piece of tape at the back. The front of the lower jaw should flop down a little to form the mouth

- Now ask participants to decorate the faces with ears, eyebrow, noses, etc. You can have piercings by using single hole punchers. They should identify a character for their puppet, e.g. health visitor, teacher, pupil, looked-after child, etc

- Ask participants to think of phrases these characters would say. Work the mouth of the puppet whilst repeating the phrases

- Ask participants to pair up and develop dialogues between puppets. Perform in front of the group and discuss their findings

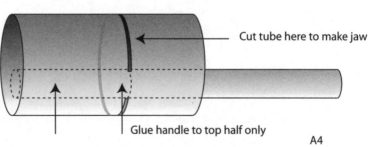

Cut tube here to make jaw

Glue handle to top half only

A4

Preparation time
Just collection of materials

Cooking time
½ hour for making puppets,
½ hour for using them

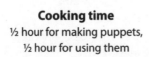

Energy level
4

Quantity
Up to 20

Puppets

These are so simple and so much fun. When working with young children you will need to pre-make the basic puppet and have a range of pre-cut features. They can be used to reflect a service, an individual or the participant themselves.

Stirabout

Ingredients

- Large sheets of thick, plain paper
- Digital camera
- Laptop
- Printer
- Magazines/photosets
- Thick pens

Method

- Identify the area you wish to explore, important places, important people, things I worry about, etc

- Let participants take photos of each other and put them on the laptop. They can then play/edit them until they are happy with the results. Print them off

- Ask the participants to place their photos on the sheet and then create a collage using the materials, writing, drawing, thinking about the chosen area

- If desired share the results and scan them into the computer at a later date

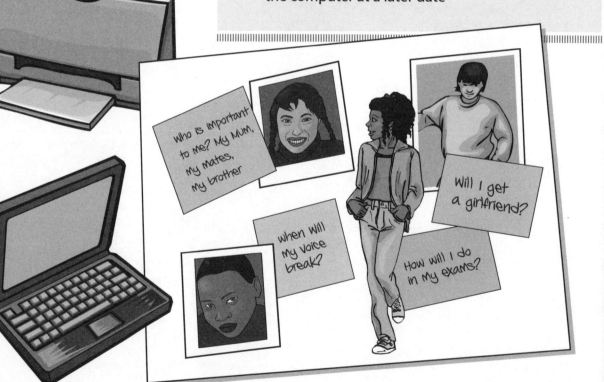

Who is important to me? My Mum, my mates, my brother

Will I get a girlfriend?

When will my voice break?

How will I do in my exams?

Preparation time
Collection of magazines

Cooking time
30 minutes

Energy level
6

Quantity
10–15

Stirabout

Children of all ages have responded well to this as it includes work on a computer! It can also be used to reflect a service, with images of that service and participants responses to it. As a baseline assessment and final evaluation it can be valuable too, the participant having an initial image of themselves and their skills and then having a final image at the end of a project, identifying their new skills.

Telescopes

Ingredients

- Tubes from kitchen rolls, cling film, foil, etc. They should be varying widths

- If tubes are difficult to obtain use card rolled into tubes

- Small circles of OHP acetates that will cover the ends of the telescope

- OHP pens of different colours

- Tape

- Scissors

- Lollipop sticks

- Small torches (optional)

Method

- Ask participants to construct telescopes from the tubes. Try and use at least 3 segments that slot into each other. Secure them with tape

- Ask participants to cut a slit into the wide end of their telescope so that the acetate circles can slot into them

- Give participants a selection of acetate circles and identify the area you wish them to focus on – e.g. where they feel most/least supported, etc. Try and get a positive and a negative

- Ask them to draw images of each of these places on the acetates and attach a lolly stick to them to provide a 'handle'. There should be two images per person reflecting positive and negative aspects of the chosen area

- Place the images into the end of the telescopes and look towards a light

- You can also shine torches through the telescope so you can project the images onto walls or screens, etc

- Ask participants to share images. Discuss

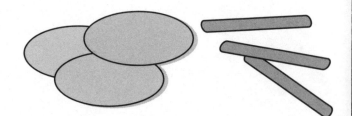

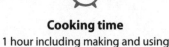		
Preparation time	**Cooking time**	**Energy level**	**Quantity**
Collection of materials	1 hour including making and using	5	Up to 30

Telescopes

This works with 9 year olds upwards and if you can manage to put a cheap plastic magnifying lens at the end of these the projected image works better.

The telescopes can be used as part of an ongoing evaluation showing how the service/individual has progressed.

Wire person (part 1)

Ingredients

- Chicken wire (the stronger ones tend to be better)
- Wire cutters
- Newspaper (lots)
- PVA (lots)
- Square base board, about 30–40 cm square
- Plasticine/modelling clay
- Luggage tags/small card pieces
- Pipe cleaners
- Acrylic paints/spray paints
- Strong staple gun or 1 inch nails

Method

- This involves making a 3-dimensional figure of a person, about 1 metre high

- First make the body by rolling a sheet of chicken wire, about 50 cm high and 1 metre wide. Secure with wire pieces. You will need to squash the top together to form a shoulder shape and tuck the bottom under so you have something to attach the legs to

- Next create the legs. The legs need to be tubes of wire about 50 cm long and wide enough so that when put together they approximately equal the width of the body. You need to bend and squash the bottoms over to create feet (about 10 cm long). Attach these to the body with wire, it is better to 'stitch' them all the way around to the base of the body with the wire

- Create the arms in the same way. You may wish to model them a little so they have a slight bend. Attach at the shoulders. It does not matter at this stage if it looks a little shoddy as it will be covered with papier mache

(Continued in part 2)

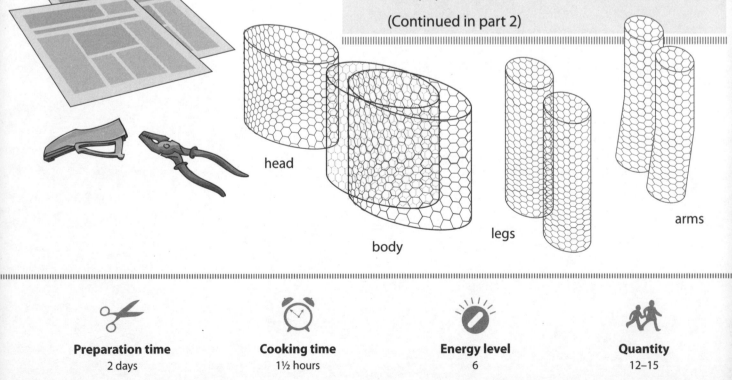

head

body

legs

arms

Preparation time	Cooking time	Energy level	Quantity
2 days	1½ hours	6	12–15

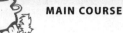

Wire person (part 2)

Method (continued)

- Next is the head. It is easier to make a tube and squash it into a kind of rectangle that is about 25 cm across and 30 cm high. Press the top together and you have a vague 'Bart Simpson' shape. Cut and fold the bottom under and attach to the top of the body

- Now attach the whole figure to the base board by stapling its feet! If you are having problems keeping it upright you may need to use an upright pole and attach the figure to that for extra support

- Cut a square door in the figure's belly and a square door/flap at the side of its head where the ear would be

- This is now the messy bit! Cover the whole thing in at least 3 layers of papier mache. Make sure any sharp edges are covered. Build up the features with extra paper/card/pulp

- When it is dry you can paint and decorate it

- Ask participants to think of what makes them happy/healthy/fit/sad/ and ask them to draw or make models/images of these and place them inside the figure's head or body. The latter is dependent on whether it is something that is heard/thought or something that we need to physically do/eat, etc

- When you have finished take out the contents and discuss as a group

This is a very long winded recipe but you can use the results time and time again so it is worth it in the long run – honest!!

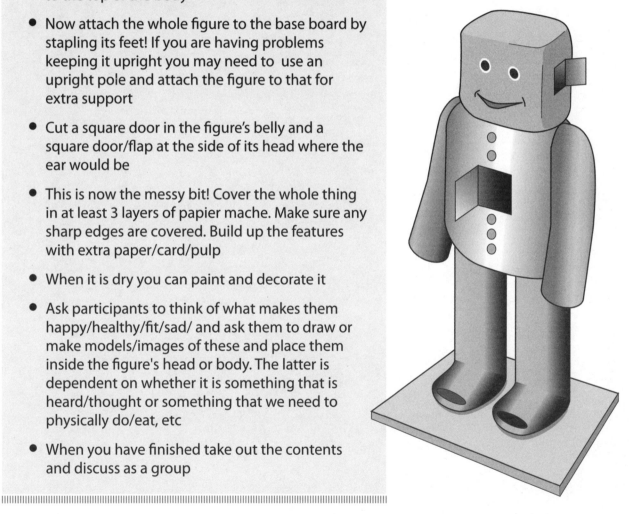

		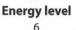	
Preparation time	**Cooking time**	**Energy level**	**Quantity**
2 days	1½ hours	6	12–15

Wire person

Very young children responded extremely well to this exercise and loved 'feeding' the character their responses and ideas. It was used extremely successfully in assessing the impact of a Health Living Project and identified that not enough work had been done around dental hygiene.

Bubbles

Ingredients

- Laminator
- White paper
- White board markers (thin)
- Digital camera

Method

- Make a series of laminated speech bubbles and thought bubbles. (Thought bubbles have a series of circles leading to them, speech bubbles have the little pointy bit!)

- Ask participants to think of a subject and write comments on their speech bubbles on how that subject is perceived by others. On the thought bubbles they should write down what they actually think of it

- Take photos of them holding the bubbles – discuss findings

- Templates for this exercise are available in the 'Ingredients' section of the Cookbook

Preparation time
30 minutes

Cooking time
15 to 30 minutes,
depending on the group

Energy level
8

Quantity
Up to 30

Bubbles

This exercise is often used as an 'add on' to some of the others and has been used in conference settings, members having their photograph taken with their responses to the conference written on the bubbles.

Images can be used if writing is an issue for participants.

Journeys

Ingredients

- Large roll of white paper, lining paper will do
- Cutouts of feet, two for each participant
- Felt tips
- Blue Tac

Method

- Roll out a large section of the paper and secure it to a wall or on the floor. Draw a path upon it

- Ask participants to identify aspirations/objectives they want to achieve. They should draw images at the end of the path

- On their footprints they should write how they are going to achieve them and place them on the 'path' in relation to when they think they might accomplish them – a kind of time-line

- This can also be used to explore aspirations for services and effectiveness of individual workshops etc. The feet can act as indicators in assessing how closely certain objectives have been hit or missed!

- Templates for this exercise are available in the 'Ingredients' section of the Cookbook

Preparation time
30 minutes

Cooking time
15 minutes

Energy level
7

Quantity
30

Journeys

This has been a very well received and useful exercise with children of a variety of ages.

It can be adapted for personal evaluation with a 'concertina' of paper being kept in a folder to mark an individual's journey through a service.

It can also be adapted in other ways with templates of football boots and goals, basketballs and nets, etc.

Picture this

Ingredients

- Huge selection of laminated images
- Flip charts
- Pens
- Camera
- Paper

Method

- Ideal for starting discussion. Ask participants to choose an area and then use the images to show what they feel about it. The images can be used as metaphors. Images should be small enough to create a flip-chart sized collage

- Have a scribe in the group/groups so they can record comments

- Photograph results. Discuss

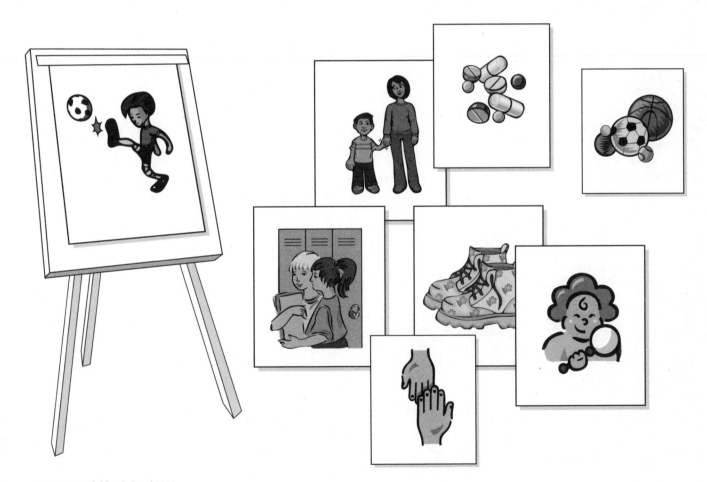

© Coventry Children's Fund 2005

Preparation time
1+ hours as it involves
a lot of collection of varied images.

Cooking time
About ½ hour

Energy level
6

Quantity
Up to 25

45

Picture this

This is a simple, non-threatening way of starting or finishing a session. Participants are made to feel less exposed and are therefore more likely to be open in their responses. Very young children can use this exercise successfully too. Pre-made images of activities or aspects of a service can be used.

PUDDING

Thermoevaluator

Ingredients

- Two pieces of A1 mounting board – white
- Felt tip pens
- Red Post-its or pieces of paper
- Strong tape

Method

- Tape the two pieces of board together on one side so that they can fold back for easier transport
- Onto one side draw a giant thermometer. Make sure you leave enough space around the outside to write in the 'temperatures'
- The lower temperature should denote coldness /uninspiring/dislike
- The middle should denote warmth/OK/reasonable
- The top should denote heat/great/inspiring
- Choose a subject and ask participants to think of a part of it, e.g. school lessons. They should write comments about these and place them where they feel they should go on the thermometer. Continue
- Take photos of the results
- Templates for this exercise are available in the 'Ingredients' section of the Cookbook

Preparation time
30 minutes

Cooking time
15 minutes

Energy level
7

Quantity
15

Thermoevaluator

This is really an upright version of the 'Targets' and again can be used as an alternative to the '1–5 scale.'

PUDDING

Webs

Ingredients

- Large ball of string
- Ways of attaching string to walls/windows
- Strips of different coloured paper
- Luggage tags
- Beads/feathers/sequins
- Pipe cleaners
- String/twine
- If pre-making webs a piece of board 1 metre square

Method

- Construct a web in the room or on a piece of board. You can either make it with a series of spokes coming out and then concentric circles or a spiral coming out from the centre

- Ask participants to think of an area in their life, e.g. home, and write their desires about this area on the luggage tags (they can use symbols if they desire)

- Ask them to decorate the web with the materials and hang them on the web. Photograph results and discuss

- If you wish you can use the web as a target with the participants placing desires/comments of what they most want/liked near the centre and least want/liked toward the outer edge

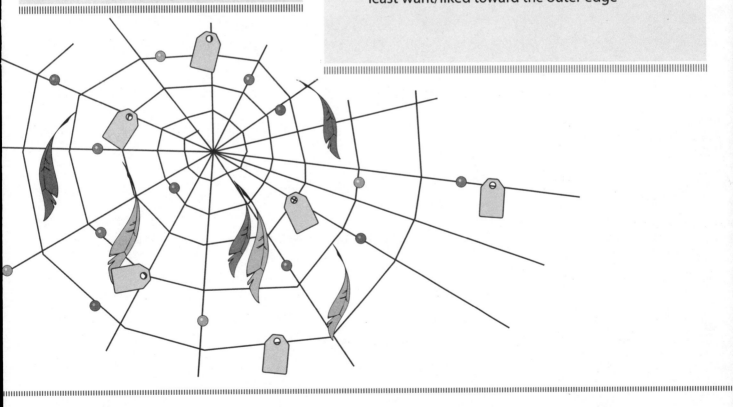

Preparation time
If doing pre-made webs
about 30 minutes

Cooking time
15 to 20 minutes

Energy level
6

Quantity
Dependent on number of
webs and size – up to 30

Webs

This is a three-dimensional version of the target and can be used as such. However, you can also section it into quarters that can then represent aspects of a service. In this way you can collect a lot of data from one exercise.

Visually the finished web is stunning; however, a certain degree of dexterity is needed for threading the buttons and decorating the labels.

Presentation

Ingredients

Presentation of findings is a very important part of the whole evaluation process and while service providers may be happy with dry, stale reports, young people may want something a little more spicy. What follows are some ideas of how you can present your findings to the young people and how they can present them to service providers. None of it involves spun sugar you will be pleased to hear!

Pockets

Pockets can be created using fabric (canvas that is then decorated with fabric paints, glitter, feathers, etc), gardening plastic glued or stitched together, by sticking paper bags onto a backing or by simply using a series of envelopes stuck onto card. You can even make something like a fisherman's jacket with the pockets stuffed to give to your service provider – great publicity shot! The pockets can be filled with findings, photos, comments and anything else that you or the children think is relevant – perhaps audio tapes of them chanting the findings that were most important to them. The possibilities are endless – go play!

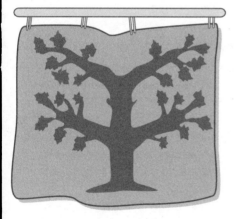

Trees

Another way of presenting and displaying findings is by attaching them to fabric trees/cardboard trees/wire trees. The branches can represent different areas of your research and you can use paper leaves, or fabric ones upon which to attach objects or fruits of your labour. The leaves could have pockets in if you wanted or there could be pockets in the branches to place tapes and photos. Again the possibilities are endless. You could do a whole piece on the seed that you want to start with (short term objectives) based on your findings, and then where you and the children would like the results to lead to – a forest perhaps! – go water!

Projections

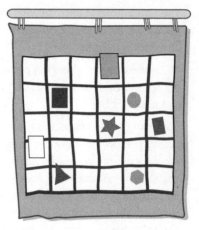

This is a really accessible way of presenting findings to service providers using children's art work and words. Have children (with this you can use the work of very young children too) draw images of their findings onto OHP sheets. Ask service providers to wear a white overall (the paper sort used for decorating, with a hood) and project the findings onto the service providers. If they are unwilling to let this happen then let the children wear large white sheets and perhaps masks that represent the service providers and project the images onto them. Choral refrains can be used to highlight the main findings. The children call them out and the service providers repeat.

Katrice Horsley would like to acknowledge Jim Morris for this idea

The Virtual Cookbook

The Evaluator's Cookbook has presented twenty-six techniques for involving children and young people in research and evaluation. Most rely on using discarded items, junk materials or none at all. As such, the approach has been distinctly 'low-tech'. Yet the exercises used can be amended and redesigned using 'high technology'. This final section offers four examples of interactive I.T. based evaluation tools which draw on the more arts-based approaches described so far.

The O-meters

The Smile-ometer and Speedometer are variations on a very familiar technique for evaluating a particular service – or session – with children and young people

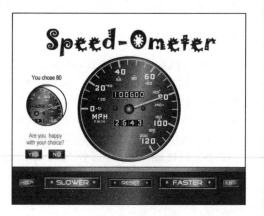

- Smile-ometer – how happy or sad am I feeling?
- Speedometer – how fast do you think we are going: too slow, too fast, or just about right?

Both can be used to record the individual view of a particular child or young person – or they can be aggregated to give statistically significant scores. *x* people were very happy with a service, *y* people were unhappy… and the overall score is… Again, these exercises do not tell you why participants were happy/unhappy, so time in front of the computer needs to be combined with discussions about 'why you feel that way?'/ 'why do you think we are going too fast/slow?'

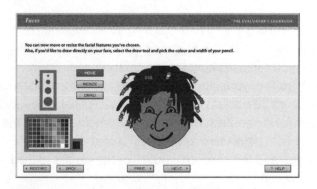

Puppets and masks

This is an electronic version of the exercise presented on page 28. Using a computer, children and young people can create 'faces' of how they feel – what they might say in public and how this might be different to what they think privately. Using computer graphics, participants can add or adjust facial features (changing the eyes, hair, skin tone, etc) to express how they feel, and add speech bubbles to explain their character and how they feel in public – and in private (see also Puppets, page 32).

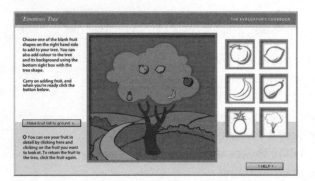

The Emotion tree

This exercise, using colour and fruits on a tree, was designed specifically for children with Asperger's Syndrome and others who find social interaction difficult. The tree can therefore be used with individual children using a computer screen. Alternatively, small groups may be asked to express their feelings and ideas using a range of different fruit symbols and colours. Findings can then be presented back to the group as a basis for further discussion. The Emotion Tree is just one variation on the feedback exercise presented on page 51.

All the exercises from the Virtual Cookbook (with full instructions) can be viewed, downloaded and used for free by visiting www.nemisys.uk.com/cookbook.

Ingredients

Templates for The Evaluator's Cookbook Exercises

Locks and keys

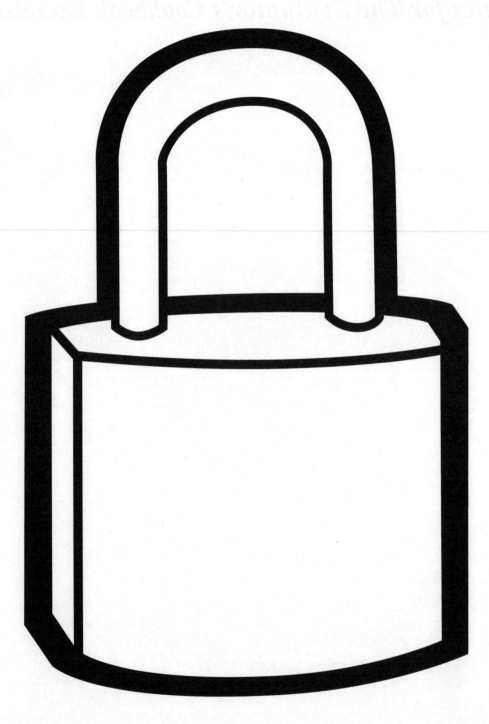

Locks and keys

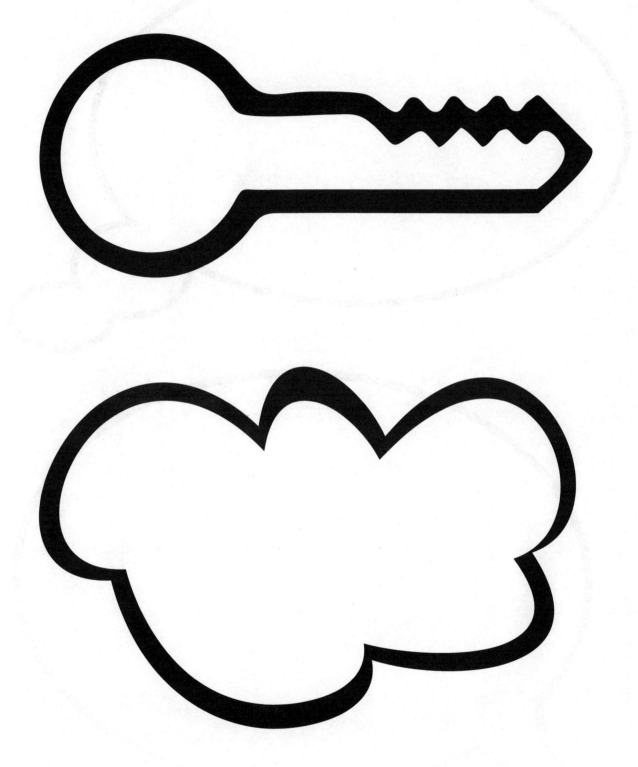

Bubbles

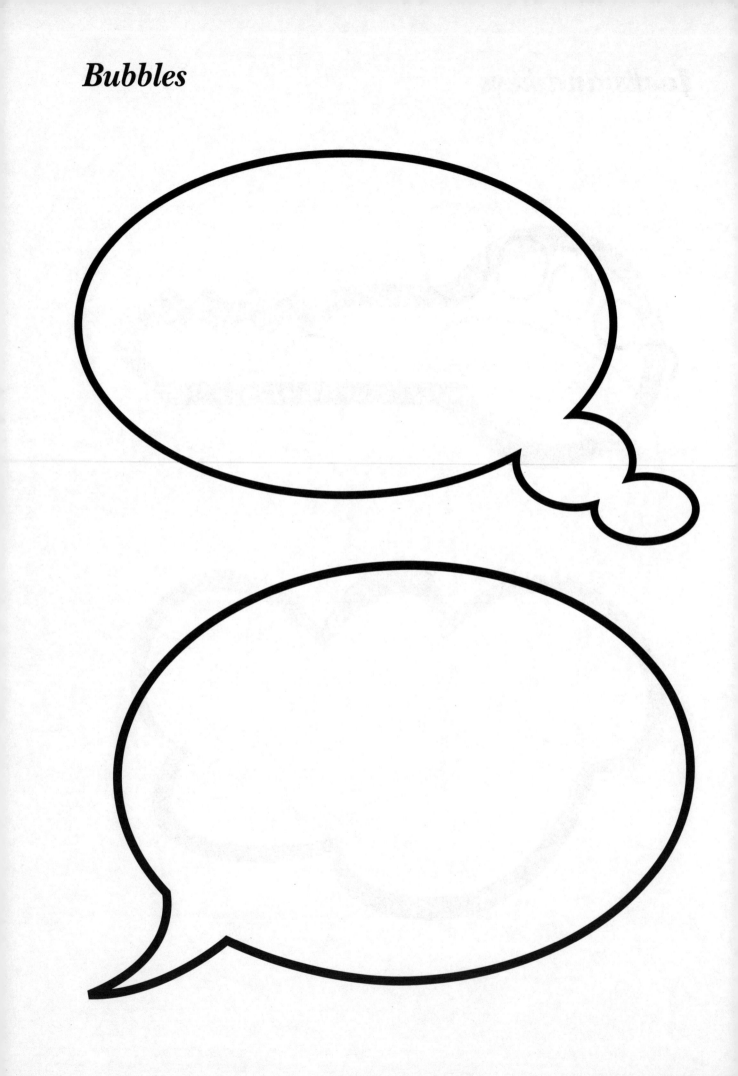

Journeys

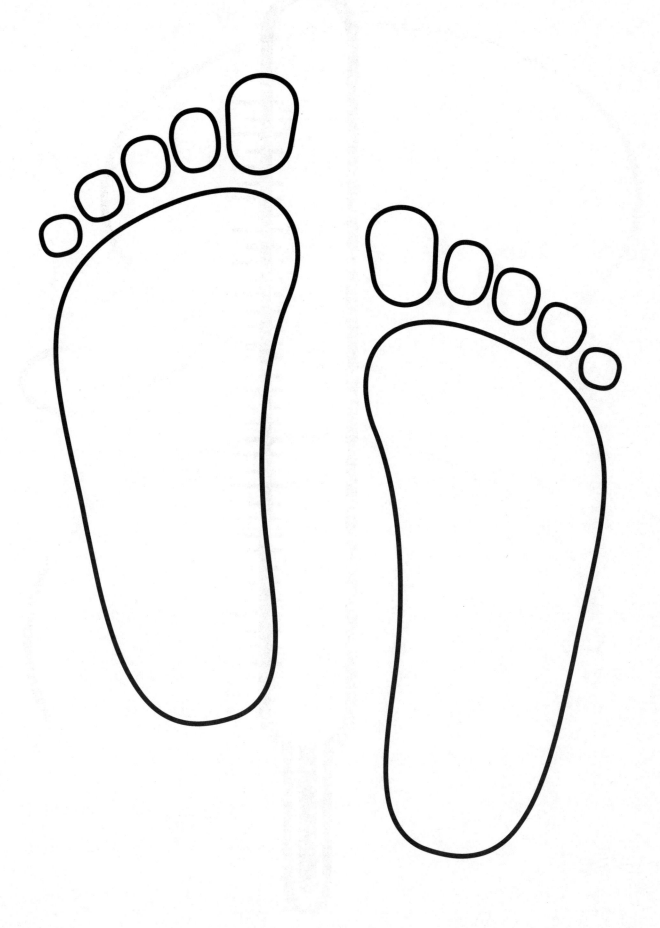

Thermoevaluator

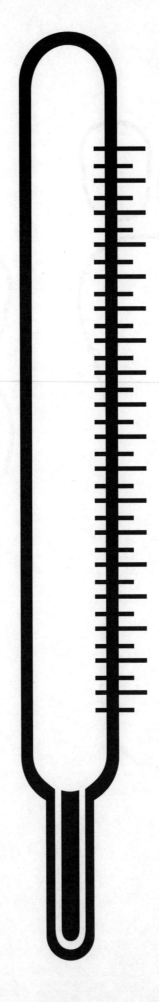